CAUSES OF PAIN ON THE BOTTOM OF YOUR FEET

UNVEILING THE CULPRITS: EXPLORING THE CAUSES OF HEEL PAIN

MARK M

Table Of Contents

INTRODUCTION ON THE CAUSES OF PAIN ON THE BOTTOM OF YOUR FEE

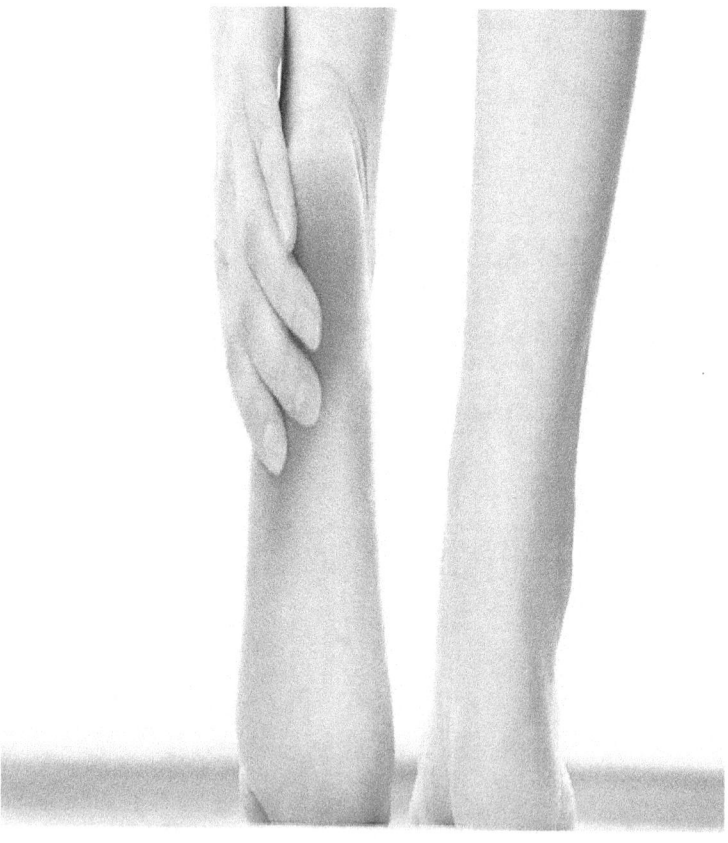

Pain on the bottom of the feet, also known as plantar pain, can result from various causes, ranging from minor issues like wearing ill-fitting shoes to more serious medical conditions. Here's an extensive overview of potential causes:

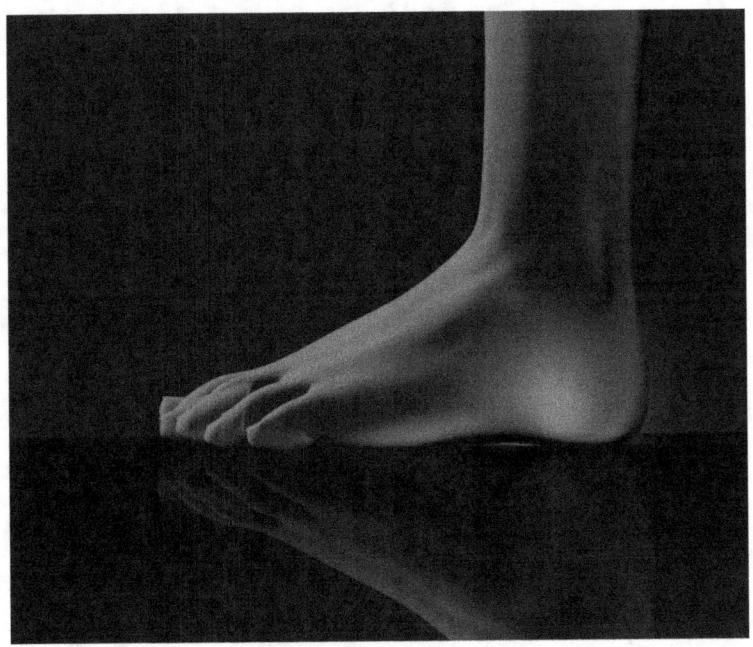

1. PLANTAR FASCIITIS

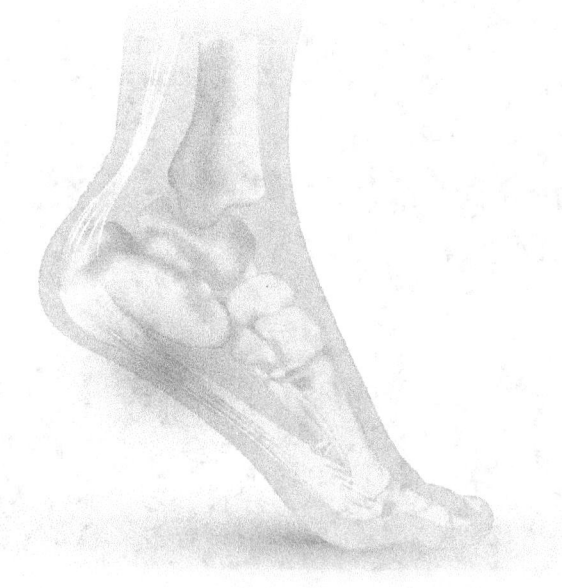

Plantar fasciitis is a common condition
characterized by inflammation of the plantar

fascia, a thick band of tissue that runs along the bottom of the foot, connecting the heel bone to the toes. This condition typically manifests as sharp or stabbing pain in the heel or arch of the foot, especially with the first steps in the morning or after prolonged periods of rest.

The plantar fascia acts as a shock absorber and supports the arch of the foot during weight-bearing activities such as walking, running, or standing. When subjected to excessive stress or repetitive strain, small tears can develop in the fascia, leading to inflammation and pain.

Several factors contribute to the development of plantar fasciitis, including:

1. Overuse or excessive strain: Activities that involve repetitive stress on the feet, such as running, jumping, or prolonged standing, can strain the plantar fascia and lead to micro-tears and inflammation.

2. Foot mechanics: Flat feet, high arches, or abnormal walking patterns (e.g., overpronation or supination) can alter the distribution of weight on the foot, placing increased stress on the plantar fascia.

3. Tight calf muscles: Tightness in the calf muscles can affect the flexibility of the Achilles tendon and the plantar fascia, increasing the risk of injury and inflammation.

4. Obesity: Excess body weight can place additional strain on the plantar fascia, increasing the risk of inflammation and pain.

5. Improper footwear: Wearing shoes with inadequate support or poor cushioning can contribute to the development of plantar fasciitis by increasing stress on the foot's tissues.

Symptoms of plantar fasciitis typically include:

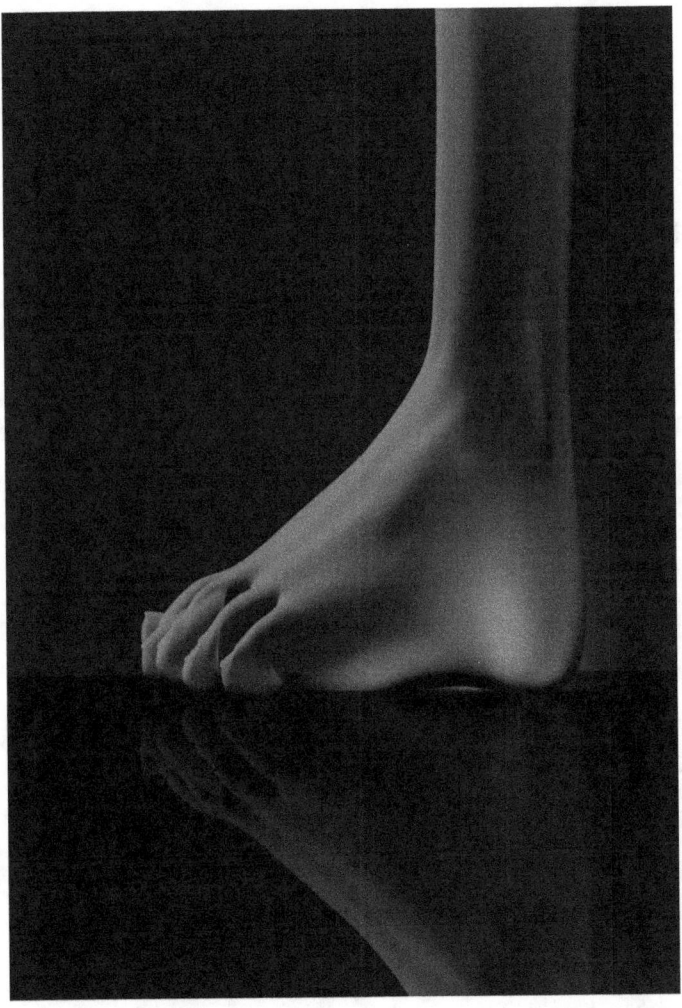

- Pain and stiffness in the bottom of the heel or along the arch of the foot, especially upon waking or after prolonged periods of rest.

- Pain that improves with activity but worsens after prolonged standing or walking.
- Tenderness and swelling in the affected area.
- Difficulty with activities that require weight-bearing on the affected foot.

Diagnosis of plantar fasciitis is usually based on a physical examination, including assessment of symptoms and the affected foot's range of motion. Imaging tests such as X-rays or ultrasound may be recommended to rule out other potential causes of heel pain and to assess the extent of tissue damage.

Treatment for plantar fasciitis typically involves a combination of conservative measures aimed at reducing pain and inflammation, improving foot mechanics, and promoting healing. These may include:

- Rest and activity modification to avoid activities that exacerbate symptoms.
- Stretching exercises to improve flexibility in the calf muscles and plantar fascia.

- Orthotic devices such as arch supports or heel cushions to provide support and relieve pressure on the plantar fascia.
- Night splints to maintain a stretched position of the plantar fascia and Achilles tendon during sleep.
- Physical therapy to strengthen the muscles of the foot and lower leg and improve biomechanical alignment.
- Nonsteroidal anti-inflammatory drugs (NSAIDs) to reduce pain and inflammation.
- Corticosteroid injections for severe or persistent pain that does not respond to conservative treatments.

In some cases, when conservative measures fail to provide relief, more invasive treatments such as extracorporeal shockwave therapy (ESWT) or surgery may be considered as a last resort.

Overall, early recognition and appropriate management of plantar fasciitis are essential for achieving a successful outcome and preventing chronic pain and disability. It's important to consult a healthcare professional for an accurate diagnosis and individualized treatment plan tailored to your specific needs.

2. METATARSALGIA

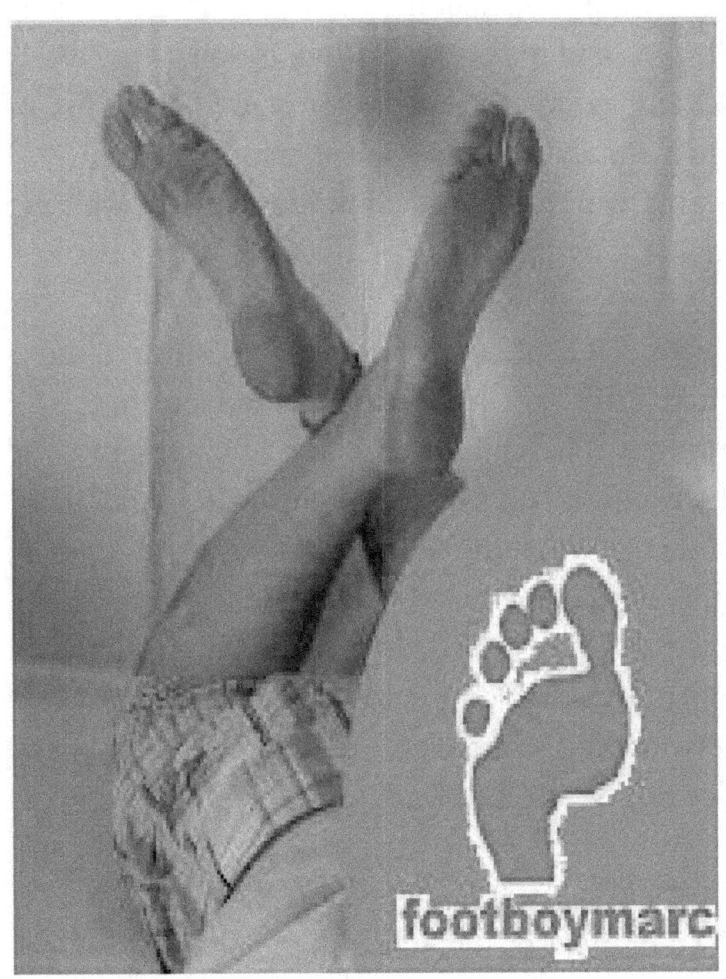

Metatarsalgia is a common foot condition characterized by pain and inflammation in the ball of the foot, specifically in the area between the toes and the arch. This condition typically develops due to excessive pressure or overuse of the metatarsal bones and surrounding tissues during weight-bearing activities such as walking, running, or standing.

The metatarsal bones are the long bones in the middle of the foot that connect the toes to the midfoot. They play a crucial role in weight distribution and propulsion during walking and running. When the metatarsal heads (the rounded ends of the metatarsal bones) are subjected to excessive stress or repetitive impact, it can lead to irritation, inflammation, and pain in the surrounding soft tissues, including the joints, ligaments, and tendons.

Several factors can contribute to the development of metatarsalgia, including:

1. Foot structure and biomechanics:
Abnormalities such as high arches, flat feet, or
uneven weight distribution can increase pressure
on the metatarsal heads, leading to irritation and
inflammation of the surrounding tissues.

2. Footwear: Wearing shoes with inadequate
support, insufficient cushioning, or narrow toe
boxes can exacerbate pressure on the ball of the
foot, contributing to the development of
metatarsalgia.

3. High-impact activities: Engaging in activities
that involve repetitive jumping, running, or
quick changes in direction can place excessive
stress on the metatarsal bones and surrounding
tissues, increasing the risk of injury and
inflammation.

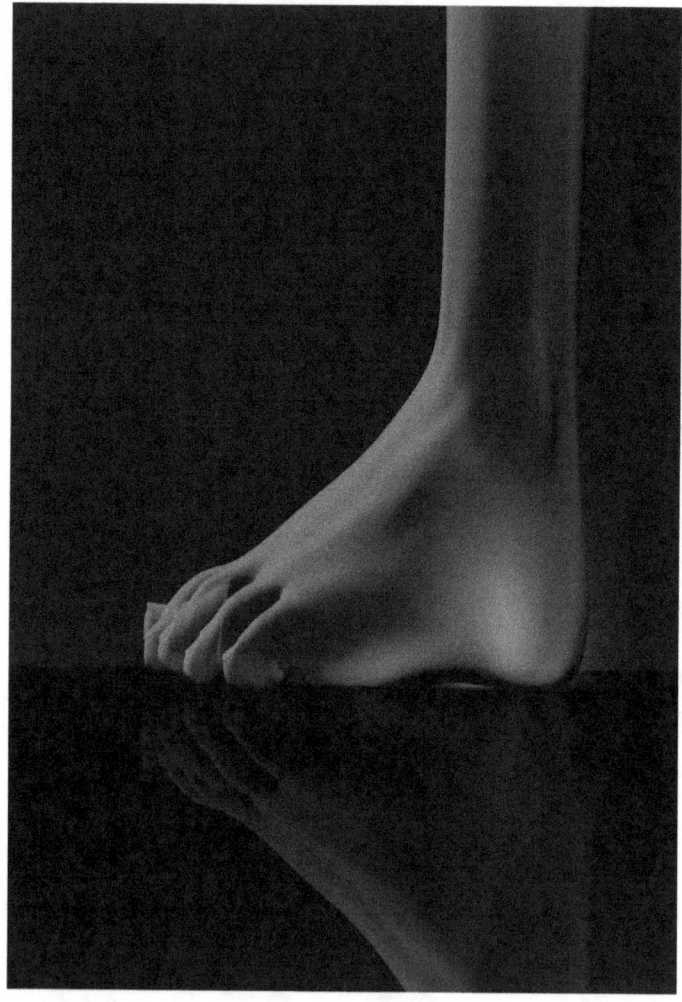

4. Foot deformities: Conditions such as
hammertoes, bunions, or Morton's toe (a
condition where the second toe is longer than the

big toe) can alter the distribution of weight on the foot, leading to increased pressure on specific metatarsal heads.

5. Obesity: Excess body weight can increase the load borne by the metatarsal bones and exacerbate pressure on the ball of the foot, contributing to the development of metatarsalgia.

Symptoms of metatarsalgia may include:

- Pain and tenderness in the ball of the foot, particularly under the heads of the metatarsal bones.
- Sharp or burning pain that worsens with weight-bearing activities and improves with rest.
- Swelling and inflammation in the affected area.
- Discomfort or numbness in the toes.
- Difficulty walking or standing for extended periods.

Diagnosis of metatarsalgia typically involves a thorough physical examination, including assessment of symptoms, foot structure, and gait analysis. Imaging tests such as X-rays or MRI scans may be ordered to rule out other potential causes of foot pain, such as stress fractures or arthritis.

Treatment for metatarsalgia usually involves a combination of conservative measures aimed at reducing pain and inflammation, improving foot mechanics, and preventing recurrence. These may include:

- Rest and activity modification to avoid activities that exacerbate symptoms.
- Ice therapy to reduce pain and inflammation in the affected area.
- Padding or orthotic devices to cushion and support the metatarsal heads and redistribute pressure on the foot.
- Proper footwear with adequate support, cushioning, and roomy toe boxes to accommodate the shape of the foot and reduce pressure on the ball of the foot.

- Stretching and strengthening exercises to improve foot flexibility, muscle strength, and biomechanical alignment.
- Nonsteroidal anti-inflammatory drugs (NSAIDs) to relieve pain and inflammation.
- Corticosteroid injections for severe or persistent pain that does not respond to conservative treatments.
- Physical therapy to address underlying biomechanical issues and improve gait mechanics.

In some cases, when conservative measures fail to provide relief, surgical intervention may be considered to correct structural abnormalities, such as bunions or hammertoes, that contribute to metatarsalgia.

Overall, early recognition and appropriate management of metatarsalgia are essential for relieving pain, improving function, and preventing long-term complications. It's important to consult a healthcare professional for an accurate diagnosis and individualized treatment plan tailored to your specific needs.

3. Heel spurs

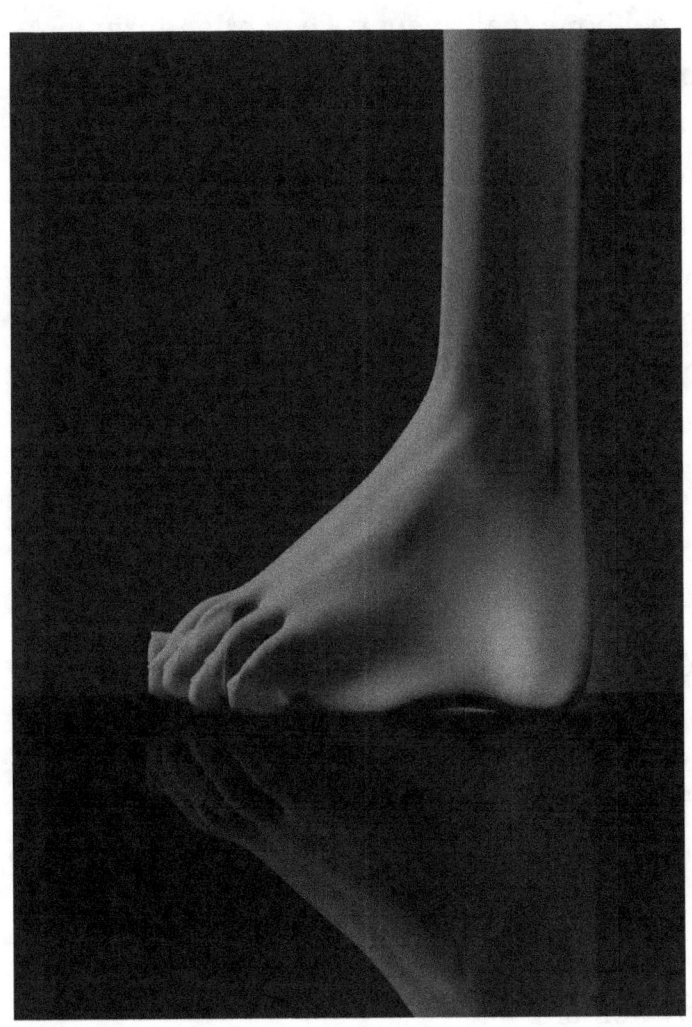

Heel spurs, also known as calcaneal spurs, are bony growths that develop on the underside of the heel bone (calcaneus). They often form in response to repetitive stress or tension on the plantar fascia, a thick band of tissue that runs along the bottom of the foot, connecting the heel bone to the toes. While heel spurs themselves may not necessarily cause pain, they can contribute to the development of conditions such as plantar fasciitis or Achilles tendonitis, which can result in heel pain and discomfort.

Here's a detailed overview of heel spurs:

1. Formation: Heel spurs typically develop over time in response to ongoing stress or tension on the plantar fascia, which may occur due to activities such as running, walking, or standing for long periods. The body's natural response to this stress is to deposit calcium at the point where the plantar fascia attaches to the heel bone, leading to the formation of a bony protrusion or spur.

2. Causes: Several factors can contribute to the development of heel spurs, including:

- Plantar fasciitis: Chronic inflammation and irritation of the plantar fascia can lead to the formation of heel spurs.

- Poor foot mechanics: Abnormalities in foot structure or biomechanics, such as flat feet, high arches, or overpronation, can increase stress on the plantar fascia and heel bone, predisposing individuals to heel spurs.

- Excessive weight: Carrying excess body weight can place additional strain on the plantar fascia and heel bone, increasing the risk of heel spur formation.

- Tight calf muscles: Reduced flexibility in the calf muscles can alter the mechanics of the foot and increase tension on the plantar fascia, contributing to heel spur development.

- Certain activities: Participating in high-impact activities or repetitive movements that strain the plantar fascia, such as running or jumping, can increase the likelihood of developing heel spurs.

3. Symptoms: Heel spurs themselves may not cause symptoms in all cases. However, they can contribute to heel pain, especially when associated with conditions such as plantar fasciitis. Common symptoms of heel spurs may include:

- Sharp or stabbing pain in the bottom of the heel, particularly with the first steps in the morning or after periods of rest.

- Pain that improves with activity but worsens with prolonged standing or walking.

- Tenderness and inflammation in the affected area.

- Discomfort or aching sensation in the heel during weight-bearing activities.

4. Diagnosis: Heel spurs are often diagnosed based on a combination of clinical evaluation, medical history, and imaging studies. X-rays are commonly used to visualize the bony growth and assess its size and location. Magnetic resonance imaging (MRI) or ultrasound may also be recommended in certain cases to evaluate soft tissue structures such as the plantar fascia.

5. Treatment: Treatment for heel spurs aims to alleviate symptoms, reduce inflammation, and address underlying contributing factors. Depending on the severity of symptoms and individual circumstances, treatment options may include:

- Rest and activity modification to avoid aggravating activities.

- Ice therapy to reduce pain and inflammation in the affected area.

- Stretching exercises to improve flexibility in the calf muscles and plantar fascia.

- Orthotic devices such as heel pads, arch supports, or custom-made shoe inserts to provide cushioning and support and relieve pressure on the heel.

- Nonsteroidal anti-inflammatory drugs (NSAIDs) to alleviate pain and inflammation.

- Physical therapy to strengthen the muscles of the foot and lower leg and improve biomechanical alignment.

- Corticosteroid injections for severe or persistent pain that does not respond to conservative measures.

- Extracorporeal shockwave therapy (ESWT) to promote tissue healing and reduce pain.

- Surgery may be considered in rare cases when conservative treatments fail to provide relief, and symptoms persist despite other interventions. Surgical options may include releasing the plantar fascia or removing the heel spur.

the management of heel spurs typically involves a comprehensive approach that addresses both the symptoms and underlying contributing factors. It's important for individuals experiencing heel pain to seek evaluation and guidance from a healthcare professional for an accurate diagnosis and personalized treatment plan. Early intervention can help alleviate symptoms, prevent complications, and improve overall foot health and function.

4. STRESS FRACTURES

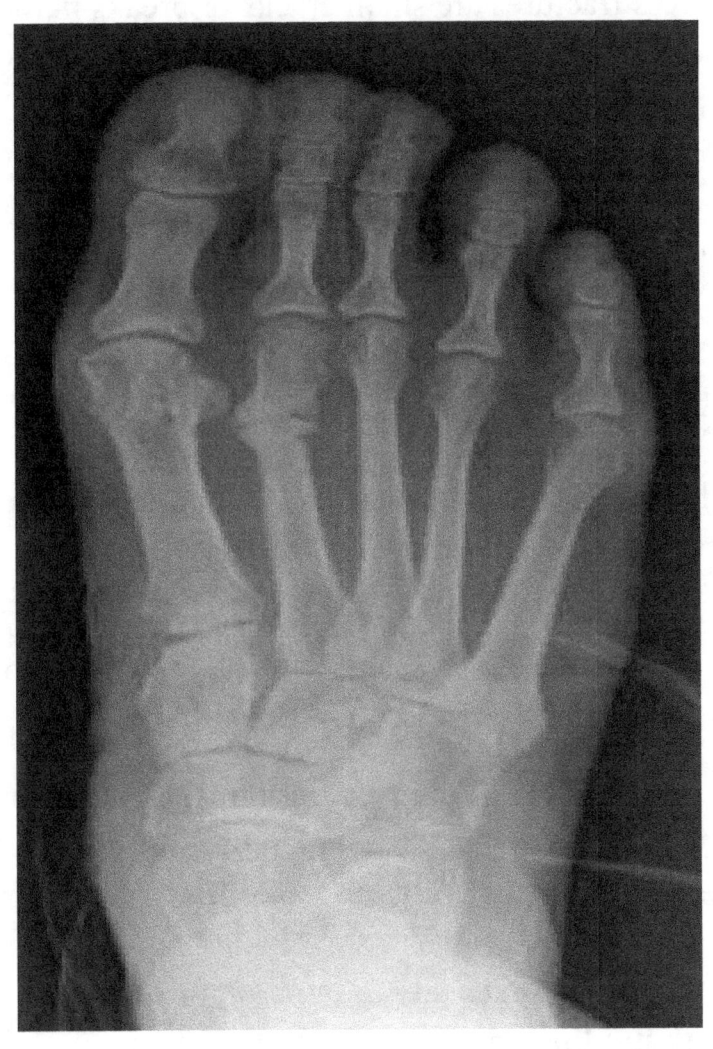

Stress fractures are small cracks or breaks in the bone that result from repetitive stress or overuse, typically caused by activities such as running, jumping, or dancing. Unlike acute fractures that occur suddenly due to a single traumatic event, stress fractures develop gradually over time as a result of repeated mechanical loading and inadequate rest for the affected bone. These fractures commonly occur in weight-bearing bones of the lower extremities, such as the shinbone (tibia), metatarsals (foot bones), or the bones of the ankle and lower leg.

Here's an extremely detailed overview of stress fractures:

1. Mechanism of Injury: Stress fractures develop when the repetitive application of force on a bone exceeds its ability to repair itself. This can occur due to various factors, including:
   - Increased intensity or duration of physical activity: Engaging in high-impact or

weight-bearing activities without proper conditioning or gradual progression can overload the bones and lead to stress fractures.

- Changes in training surface: Transitioning to harder surfaces or uneven terrain can increase the stress on the bones and predispose individuals to stress fractures.

- Poor biomechanics: Abnormalities in foot structure, gait mechanics, or muscle imbalances can alter the distribution of forces on the bones, increasing the risk of stress fractures.

- Inadequate footwear: Wearing shoes that lack sufficient cushioning, support, or shock absorption can increase the impact forces transmitted to the bones, contributing to stress fractures.

- Nutritional deficiencies: Inadequate intake of calcium, vitamin D, or other nutrients essential for bone health can impair the bone's ability to withstand repetitive stress and repair microdamage.

2. Types of Stress Fractures: Stress fractures can be classified based on their location, severity, and underlying cause. Common types include:

- Metatarsal stress fractures: Small cracks in the long bones of the foot, often caused by repetitive impact from activities like running or jumping.

- Tibial stress fractures: Fractures of the shinbone (tibia), which can occur in the lower or upper portion of the bone and are frequently seen in runners and military personnel.

- Femoral neck stress fractures: Hairline fractures in the neck of the femur (thigh bone), commonly seen in athletes involved in high-impact sports such as distance running or gymnastics.

- Navicular stress fractures: Fractures of the navicular bone in the midfoot, typically seen in athletes with high arches or those engaged in activities that involve repetitive jumping or cutting motions.

3. Symptoms: The symptoms of stress fractures can vary depending on the location and severity

of the injury. Common signs and symptoms may include:

- Localized pain that worsens with weight-bearing activities and improves with rest.
- Tenderness, swelling, or bruising over the affected bone.
- Pain that is reproducible with palpation or specific movements.
- Increased discomfort during or after physical activity, with pain often described as dull, achy, or throbbing.
- Difficulty bearing weight on the affected limb or performing activities of daily living.

4. Diagnosis: Diagnosing stress fractures typically involves a combination of clinical evaluation, medical history, imaging studies, and diagnostic tests. Common methods used to diagnose stress fractures include:

- Physical examination: A healthcare professional may assess the affected area for signs of tenderness, swelling, or deformity and inquire about the onset and nature of symptoms.

- Imaging studies: X-rays are commonly used to detect stress fractures, although they may not always be visible in the early stages. Magnetic resonance imaging (MRI) or bone scans may be recommended for a more sensitive evaluation of bone microdamage.

- Bone scan: A nuclear medicine imaging test that uses a small amount of radioactive tracer to detect areas of increased bone turnover or inflammation, which may indicate the presence of a stress fracture.

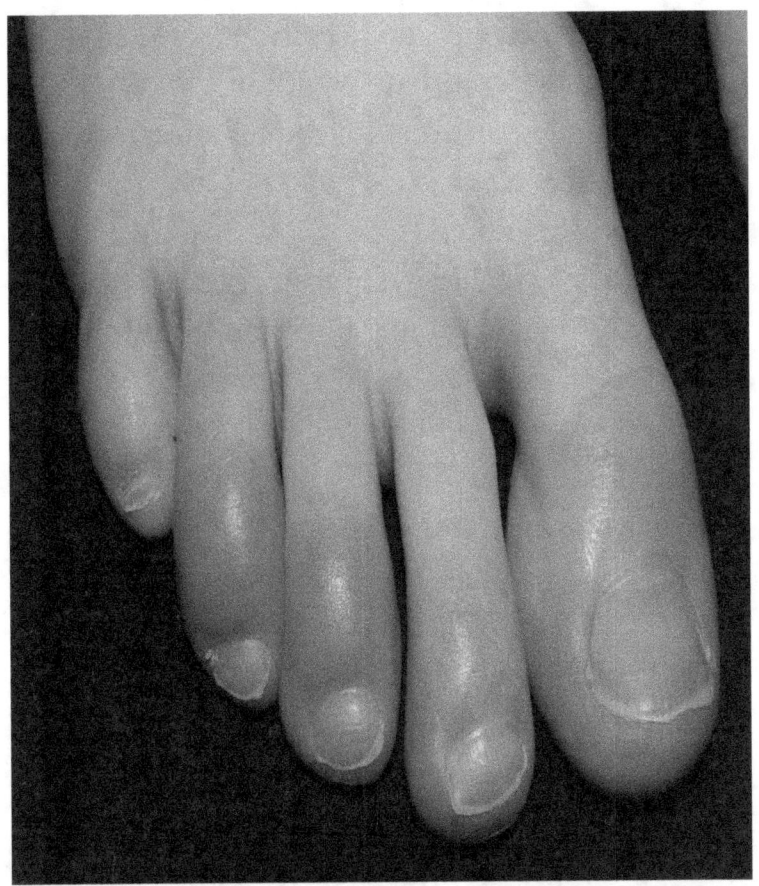

5. Treatment: Treatment for stress fractures aims to relieve pain, promote healing, and prevent complications. Depending on the severity and location of the fracture, treatment options may include:

- Rest and activity modification: Avoiding activities that exacerbate symptoms and providing adequate rest for the affected bone to heal.

- Immobilization: Using a cast, walking boot, or crutches to reduce weight-bearing on the affected limb and protect the bone from further injury.

- Ice therapy: Applying ice packs to the affected area to reduce pain and inflammation.

- Pain management: Over-the-counter pain medications such as acetaminophen or nonsteroidal anti-inflammatory drugs (NSAIDs) may be used to alleviate discomfort.

- Orthotic devices: Custom orthotics or supportive footwear may be prescribed to help distribute pressure more evenly across the foot and reduce stress on the affected bone.

- Physical therapy: Gradual rehabilitation exercises to improve strength, flexibility, and biomechanics, as well as to facilitate a safe return to activity.

- Extracorporeal shock wave therapy (ESWT): A noninvasive treatment modality that uses shock waves to stimulate healing and promote bone regeneration in chronic or nonhealing stress fractures.

- Surgical intervention: In rare cases of severe or nonhealing stress fractures, surgery may be necessary to stabilize the bone and facilitate healing. This may involve internal fixation with screws, plates, or pins to realign the fractured fragments.

6. Complications and Prognosis: Without appropriate treatment and rest, stress fractures can progress to more severe injuries, such as complete fractures or delayed union. Chronic or recurrent stress fractures may also increase the risk of long-term complications, including persistent pain, reduced bone density, or stress fracture recurrence. However, with prompt diagnosis and appropriate management, most stress fractures heal well with conservative measures, and individuals can typically return to their previous level of activity within a few weeks to months.

stress fractures are common overuse injuries characterized by small cracks or breaks in the bone due to repetitive stress. Early recognition, proper diagnosis, and timely intervention are essential for effective treatment and prevention of complications. Individuals experiencing symptoms suggestive of a stress fracture should seek evaluation and guidance from a healthcare professional for an accurate diagnosis and individualized treatment plan.

5. NEUROPATHY

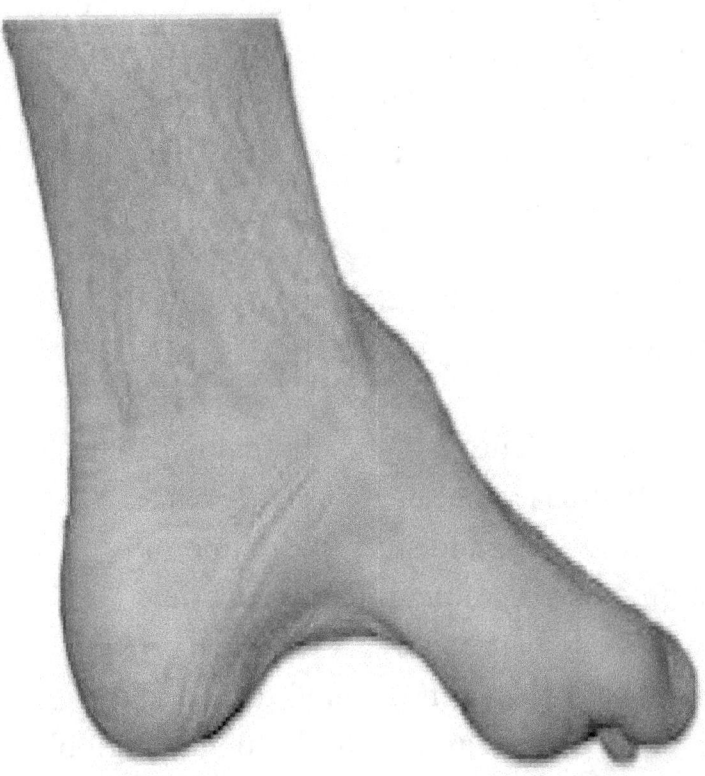

Neuropathy, also known as peripheral neuropathy, refers to a condition characterized by damage or dysfunction of the peripheral nerves, which transmit signals between the central nervous system (brain and spinal cord)

and the rest of the body. This disruption in nerve function can lead to a wide range of symptoms, including pain, numbness, tingling, weakness, and changes in sensation, often affecting the hands and feet. Neuropathy can result from various underlying causes and may be acute or chronic in nature.

Here's an extremely detailed overview of neuropathy:

1. Types of Neuropathy: Neuropathy can be classified based on the underlying cause, affected nerves, and specific symptoms. Common types of neuropathy include:
   - Diabetic neuropathy: A common complication of diabetes mellitus, characterized by nerve damage related to prolonged high blood sugar levels.
   - Peripheral neuropathy: A generalized term for nerve damage affecting the peripheral nerves outside the brain and spinal cord, often causing symptoms in the hands, feet, arms, and legs.

- Polyneuropathy: Involves damage to multiple peripheral nerves, leading to widespread symptoms such as pain, numbness, and weakness.

- Mononeuropathy: Affects a single nerve or nerve group, causing localized symptoms in a specific area of the body.

- Autonomic neuropathy: Involves damage to the nerves that control involuntary bodily functions such as heart rate, blood pressure, digestion, and bladder function.

- Hereditary neuropathy: Genetic conditions that cause nerve damage, such as Charcot-Marie-Tooth disease.

2. Causes of Neuropathy: Neuropathy can be caused by a wide range of factors, including:

- Diabetes mellitus: Prolonged exposure to high blood sugar levels can damage nerves throughout the body, leading to diabetic neuropathy.

- Trauma or injury: Direct physical trauma, such as fractures, crush injuries, or compression of nerves, can result in nerve damage and neuropathic symptoms.

- Infections: Viral or bacterial infections, such as shingles (herpes zoster), HIV/AIDS, Lyme disease, or leprosy, can cause neuropathy.

- Autoimmune diseases: Conditions such as rheumatoid arthritis, lupus, or Guillain-Barré syndrome involve the immune system attacking the body's own nerves, leading to nerve damage.

- Toxic substances: Exposure to certain toxins, chemicals, or medications, including chemotherapy drugs, heavy metals, or alcohol, can cause nerve damage and neuropathic symptoms.

- Nutritional deficiencies: Inadequate intake of essential nutrients such as vitamin B12, folate, or thiamine can impair nerve function and contribute to neuropathy.

- Genetic factors: Hereditary conditions or genetic mutations can predispose individuals to develop neuropathy.

3. Symptoms of Neuropathy: The symptoms of neuropathy can vary depending on the type,

location, and severity of nerve damage.
Common symptoms may include:

- Pain: Sharp, stabbing, burning, or shooting pain, often described as pins and needles or electric shocks.

- Numbness or tingling: Loss of sensation or abnormal sensations, such as tingling, prickling, or crawling sensations.

- Muscle weakness: Difficulty with fine motor skills, weakness, or muscle atrophy in the affected area.

- Sensory changes: Altered sensation, hypersensitivity to touch, temperature changes, or numbness in the hands, feet, arms, or legs.

- Loss of balance or coordination: Difficulty walking, unsteadiness, or increased risk of falls due to impaired proprioception.

- Autonomic symptoms: Symptoms affecting involuntary bodily functions, such as dizziness, lightheadedness, changes in heart rate or blood pressure, gastrointestinal disturbances, or bladder dysfunction.

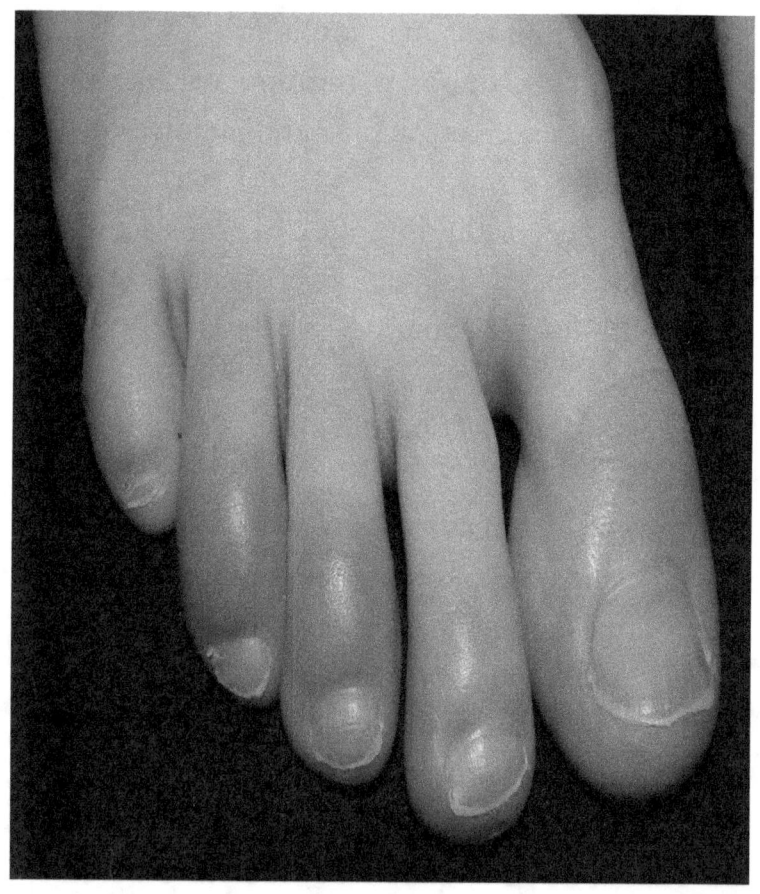

4. Diagnosis of Neuropathy: Diagnosing neuropathy typically involves a thorough medical history, physical examination, neurological assessment, and diagnostic tests.

Common methods used to diagnose neuropathy include:

- Medical history: A healthcare professional will inquire about symptoms, medical conditions, medications, family history, and potential risk factors for neuropathy.

- Physical examination: Assessment of muscle strength, reflexes, sensation, and coordination, as well as examination of the hands, feet, and other affected areas for signs of nerve damage.

- Neurological testing: Evaluation of nerve function through tests such as nerve conduction studies, electromyography (EMG), or quantitative sensory testing (QST).

- Blood tests: Laboratory tests to assess blood sugar levels, vitamin levels, kidney function, thyroid function, and other metabolic parameters that may be associated with neuropathy.

- Imaging studies: X-rays, CT scans, MRI scans, or nerve ultrasound may be used to visualize the structure of nerves and surrounding tissues and identify potential causes of neuropathy.

5. Treatment of Neuropathy: Treatment for neuropathy aims to alleviate symptoms, slow the progression of nerve damage, and address underlying causes. Depending on the type and severity of neuropathy, treatment options may include:

- Pain management: Medications such as analgesics, nonsteroidal anti-inflammatory drugs (NSAIDs), antidepressants, anticonvulsants, or topical agents may be prescribed to manage neuropathic pain.

- Blood sugar control: Tight control of blood glucose levels is essential for individuals with diabetic neuropathy to prevent further nerve damage.

- Physical therapy: Exercises to improve strength, flexibility, balance, and gait mechanics, as well as modalities such as transcutaneous electrical nerve stimulation (TENS) or ultrasound therapy to alleviate pain and improve nerve function.

- Occupational therapy: Techniques to optimize function and independence in daily activities, ergonomic modifications, and assistive devices to compensate for sensory or motor deficits.

- Lifestyle modifications: Adopting a healthy lifestyle, including regular exercise, a balanced diet, smoking cessation, and moderation of alcohol consumption, can help manage symptoms and reduce the risk of complications.

- Nutritional supplementation: Supplementation with vitamins, minerals, or other nutrients may be recommended to address deficiencies associated with neuropathy, such as vitamin B12, folate, or alpha-lipoic acid.

- Nerve blocks or injections: Local anesthetic or corticosteroid injections may be used to provide temporary pain relief and reduce inflammation in the affected nerves.

- Alternative therapies: Complementary and alternative approaches such as acupuncture, biofeedback, relaxation techniques, or herbal supplements may be considered for symptom management in some cases.

- Surgical intervention: In rare cases of severe or refractory neuropathy, surgical procedures such as nerve decompression or neuroma excision may be performed to relieve pressure on affected nerves or remove damaged tissue.

6. Prognosis and Complications: The prognosis for neuropathy depends on various factors, including the underlying cause, severity of nerve damage, response to treatment, and adherence to lifestyle modifications. While some forms of neuropathy may improve or stabilize with appropriate management, others may progress over time and lead to chronic symptoms or complications. Complications of neuropathy may include chronic pain, sensory loss, impaired mobility, increased risk of falls or injuries, poor wound healing, foot ulcers, infections, and decreased quality of life. Early recognition, prompt diagnosis, and comprehensive management are essential for optimizing outcomes and preventing long-term complications in individuals with neuropathy.

 neuropathy is a complex and multifaceted condition characterized by damage or dysfunction of

6. ACHILLES TENDONITIS

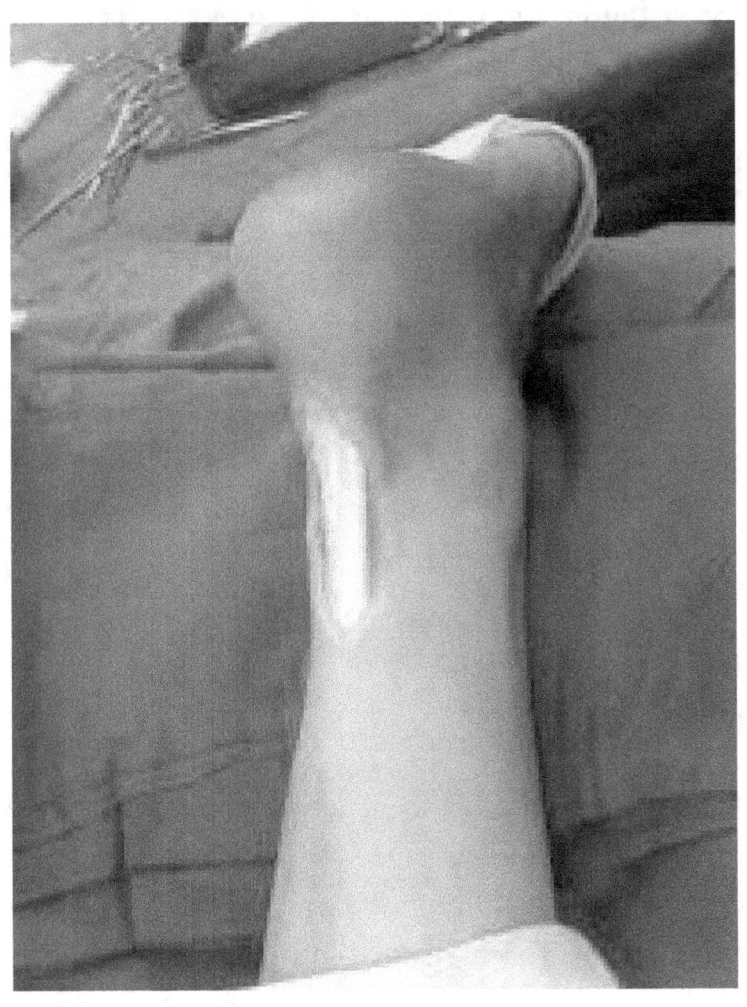

Achilles tendonitis, also known as Achilles tendinitis, is a common condition characterized by inflammation of the Achilles tendon, the large tendon that connects the calf muscles to the heel bone (calcaneus). It typically manifests as pain and stiffness in the back of the heel or lower calf, especially during physical activity or upon waking in the morning. Achilles tendonitis can range from mild discomfort to severe pain and may affect individuals of all ages, particularly those who engage in activities that place repetitive stress on the Achilles tendon, such as running, jumping, or sports involving sudden stops and starts.

Here's an extremely detailed overview of Achilles tendonitis:

1. Anatomy of the Achilles Tendon: The Achilles tendon is the strongest and largest tendon in the human body, responsible for transmitting forces from the calf muscles to the heel bone during activities such as walking, running, and jumping. It is composed of fibrous

tissue and is divided into two segments: the gastrocnemius tendon, which originates from the two heads of the calf muscle, and the soleus tendon, which arises from the deeper calf muscle. The Achilles tendon inserts into the back of the heel bone (calcaneus) and plays a crucial role in ankle movement and propulsion.

2. Causes of Achilles Tendonitis: Achilles tendonitis typically develops due to repetitive stress or overuse of the Achilles tendon, leading to microtrauma, inflammation, and degeneration of the tendon fibers. Several factors can contribute to the development of Achilles tendonitis, including:

- Overuse or sudden increase in physical activity: Engaging in activities such as running, jumping, or sports without proper conditioning or gradual progression can overload the Achilles tendon and increase the risk of injury.

- Tight calf muscles: Reduced flexibility in the calf muscles can alter the biomechanics of the ankle joint and increase stress on the Achilles tendon during movement.

- Poor footwear: Wearing shoes with inadequate support, cushioning, or stability can exacerbate stress on the Achilles tendon and contribute to the development of tendonitis.

- Biomechanical abnormalities: Abnormalities in foot structure, gait mechanics, or lower limb alignment, such as flat feet, high arches, or overpronation, can increase the risk of Achilles tendonitis.

- Age-related changes: Degenerative changes in the tendon structure and reduced blood flow to the Achilles tendon with aging can impair its ability to withstand stress and predispose individuals to tendonitis.

- Previous injury: Previous episodes of Achilles tendon injury, such as tendon strains, tears, or ruptures, can weaken the tendon and increase susceptibility to recurrent tendonitis.

3. Symptoms of Achilles Tendonitis: The symptoms of Achilles tendonitis typically develop gradually and may worsen over time with continued activity. Common signs and symptoms may include:

- Pain and stiffness in the back of the heel or lower calf, especially during physical activity or upon waking in the morning.
- Tenderness and swelling along the course of the Achilles tendon.
- Thickening or nodules within the tendon.
- Increased pain with activity that improves with rest.
- Difficulty with activities such as walking, running, or climbing stairs.
- Crepitus or creaking sensation with ankle movement in severe cases.

4. Diagnosis of Achilles Tendonitis: Diagnosing Achilles tendonitis typically involves a combination of medical history, physical examination, and diagnostic tests. Common methods used to diagnose Achilles tendonitis include:

- Medical history: A healthcare professional will inquire about symptoms, previous injuries, medical conditions, medications, and activity level.

- Physical examination: Assessment of the affected foot and ankle for signs of swelling, tenderness, warmth, thickening of the Achilles tendon, and range of motion.

- Palpation: Gentle palpation along the course of the Achilles tendon to assess for tenderness, nodules, or thickening.

- Functional tests: Evaluation of ankle range of motion, strength, flexibility, and gait mechanics to identify biomechanical abnormalities or compensatory patterns.

- Imaging studies: X-rays may be ordered to rule out other potential causes of heel pain, such as fractures or arthritis. Ultrasound or MRI scans may be used to visualize the Achilles tendon structure, assess for signs of inflammation, degeneration, or tears, and determine the extent of tendon involvement.

5. Treatment of Achilles Tendonitis: Treatment for Achilles tendonitis aims to alleviate pain, reduce inflammation, promote healing, and prevent recurrence. Depending on the severity

and duration of symptoms, treatment options may include:

- Rest and activity modification: Avoiding activities that exacerbate symptoms and providing adequate rest for the affected tendon to heal.

- Ice therapy: Applying ice packs to the affected area for 15-20 minutes several times a day to reduce pain and inflammation.

- Eccentric strengthening exercises: Progressive loading exercises to strengthen the calf muscles and Achilles tendon and promote tissue remodeling.

- Stretching exercises: Gentle stretching of the calf muscles and Achilles tendon to improve flexibility and reduce tension.

- Orthotic devices: Heel lifts, shoe inserts, or custom orthotics may be prescribed to support the arch, reduce stress on the Achilles tendon, and correct biomechanical abnormalities.

- Nonsteroidal anti-inflammatory drugs (NSAIDs): Oral medications such as ibuprofen or naproxen may be used to alleviate pain and inflammation.

- Physical therapy: Modalities such as ultrasound, laser therapy, or electrical stimulation may be used to promote tissue healing and reduce pain. Manual therapy techniques such as massage, myofascial release, or joint mobilization may also be beneficial.

- Extracorporeal shock wave therapy (ESWT): A noninvasive treatment modality that uses shock waves to stimulate healing and reduce pain in chronic cases of Achilles tendonitis.

- Corticosteroid injections: Injections of corticosteroids may be considered for severe or refractory cases of Achilles tendonitis to reduce inflammation and pain. However, repeated injections should be avoided due to the risk of tendon weakening and rupture.

- Platelet-rich plasma (PRP) therapy: A regenerative treatment approach that involves injecting concentrated platelets from the patient's own blood into the affected tendon to promote tissue repair and regeneration.

- Surgical intervention: In rare cases of severe or chronic Achilles tendonitis that do not respond to conservative treatments, surgical procedures such as debridement, tendon repair, or tendon transfer may be necessary to address underlying pathology and restore function.

6. Complications and Prognosis: With prompt diagnosis and appropriate treatment, most cases of Achilles tendonitis resolve within a few weeks to months, and individuals can typically return to their previous level of activity. However, untreated or recurrent cases of Achilles tendonitis can lead to chronic pain, tendon degeneration, tendon thickening, tendon rupture, or long-term disability. Complications of Achilles tendonitis may include impaired mobility, decreased athletic performance, altered gait mechanics, and increased risk of secondary injuries. Early intervention, adherence to treatment recommendations, and modification of risk factors are essential for optimizing outcomes and preventing long-term complications in individuals with Achilles tendonitis.

Achilles tendonitis is a common condition characterized by inflammation of the Achilles tendon due to repetitive stress or overuse. Prompt diagnosis, conservative management, and modification of contributing factors are key to effective treatment and prevention of complications. Individuals experiencing symptoms suggestive of Achilles tendonitis should seek evaluation and guidance from a healthcare professional for an accurate diagnosis and individualized treatment plan

7. MORTON'S NEUROMA

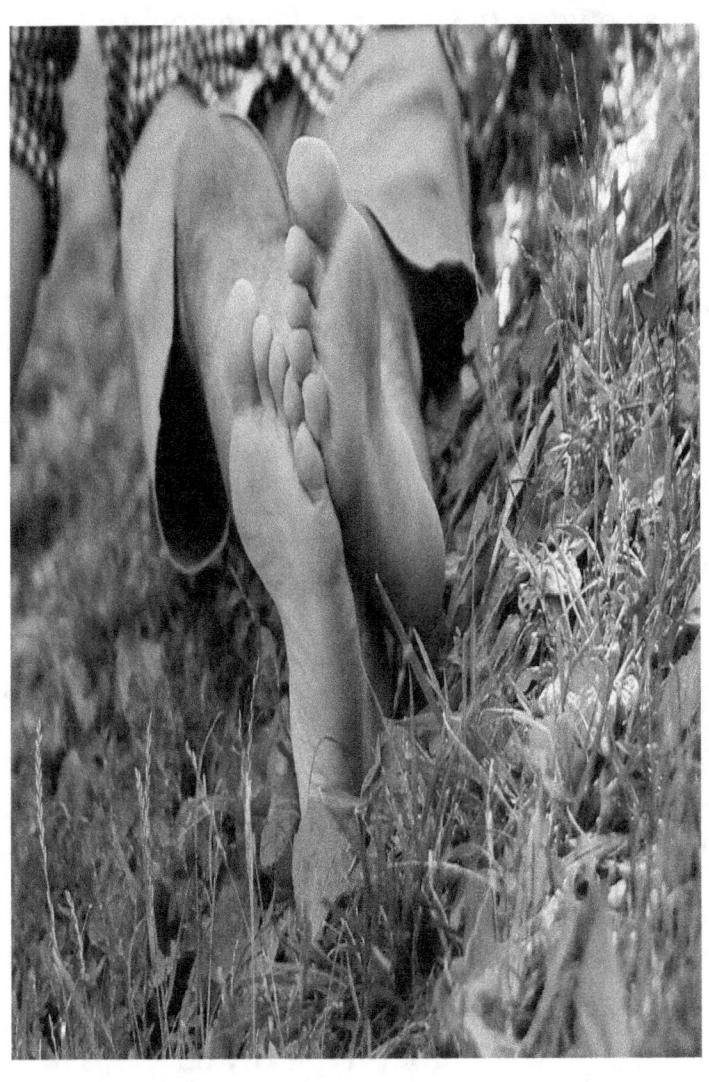

Morton's neuroma, also known as interdigital neuroma, is a painful condition that affects the nerves between the toes, most commonly between the third and fourth toes. It involves the thickening of the tissue around one of the nerves leading to the toes, which can cause sharp, burning pain, tingling, or numbness in the ball of the foot and between the toes. Morton's neuroma often develops gradually over time and can significantly impact mobility and quality of life, especially when left untreated.

Here's an extremely detailed overview of Morton's neuroma:

1. Anatomy of Morton's Neuroma: Morton's neuroma occurs at the point where the plantar digital nerve branches into the toes. This nerve is located in the ball of the foot and is responsible for providing sensation to the toes. When the nerve becomes compressed or irritated, it can lead to the formation of a neuroma, which is a noncancerous growth or thickening of nerve tissue. Morton's neuroma typically develops

between the third and fourth toes or the second and third toes, although it can occur between any of the toes.

2. Causes of Morton's Neuroma: The exact cause of Morton's neuroma is not always clear, but several factors may contribute to its development, including:

   - Footwear: Wearing tight, narrow, or high-heeled shoes can compress the toes and exacerbate pressure on the nerves, increasing the risk of neuroma formation.

   - Foot structure: Certain foot abnormalities, such as high arches, flat feet, or bunions, can alter the distribution of weight on the feet and contribute to the development of neuromas.

   - Repetitive stress: Activities that involve repetitive pressure or trauma to the ball of the foot, such as running, jumping, or wearing tight-fitting shoes for extended periods, can irritate the nerves and lead to neuroma formation.

- Injury: Trauma or injury to the foot, such as stubbing the toe, can damage the nerves and predispose individuals to develop neuromas.

- Biomechanical issues: Abnormalities in gait mechanics or foot alignment, such as overpronation or supination, can increase stress on the nerves and contribute to neuroma development.

- Certain medical conditions: Conditions such as rheumatoid arthritis, diabetes, or Morton's toe (a condition where the second toe is longer than the big toe) may increase the risk of neuroma formation.

3. Symptoms of Morton's Neuroma: The symptoms of Morton's neuroma can vary in severity and may worsen over time. Common signs and symptoms may include:

- Sharp, burning pain in the ball of the foot or between the toes, typically aggravated by walking, standing, or wearing tight shoes.

- Tingling, numbness, or a feeling of "pins and needles" in the toes or the ball of the foot.

- Sensation of a lump or foreign object under the ball of the foot.

- Pain that radiates into the toes or up the foot, sometimes mimicking the symptoms of other foot conditions such as plantar fasciitis or metatarsalgia.

- Discomfort or difficulty walking or bearing weight on the affected foot.

- Relief of symptoms with rest or by removing shoes and massaging the affected area.

4. Diagnosis of Morton's Neuroma: Diagnosing Morton's neuroma typically involves a combination of medical history, physical examination, and diagnostic tests. Common methods used to diagnose Morton's neuroma include:

- Medical history: A healthcare professional will inquire about symptoms, medical conditions, footwear habits, occupation, and activity level.

- Physical examination: Assessment of the affected foot for signs of tenderness, swelling, or thickening of the nerves between the toes, as well as evaluation of foot structure, gait mechanics, and range of motion.

- Palpation: Gentle palpation of the ball of the foot or between the toes to elicit tenderness, reproduce symptoms, and identify the location of the neuroma.

- Mulder's sign: A diagnostic maneuver where the healthcare professional squeezes the metatarsal heads while simultaneously pressing on the space between the affected toes, causing a "clicking" sensation or reproducing symptoms characteristic of Morton's neuroma.

- Imaging studies: X-rays may be ordered to rule out other potential causes of foot pain, such as stress fractures or arthritis. Ultrasound or MRI scans may be used to visualize the nerves and soft tissues in the foot and confirm the presence of a neuroma.

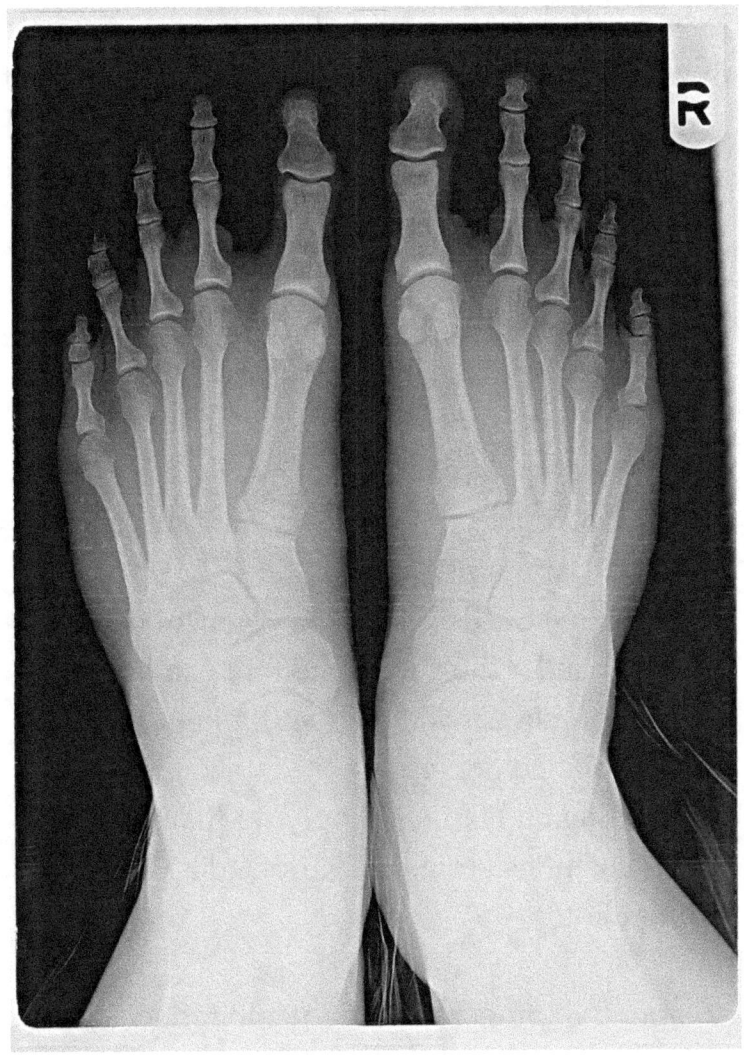

5. Treatment of Morton's Neuroma: Treatment
for Morton's neuroma aims to relieve pain,

reduce inflammation, and alleviate pressure on the affected nerves. Depending on the severity of symptoms and individual circumstances, treatment options may include:

- Footwear modifications: Switching to wider, more supportive shoes with low heels and ample room in the toe box to reduce pressure on the nerves and provide cushioning and support.

- Orthotic devices: Custom orthotic inserts or pads may be prescribed to redistribute pressure on the foot, correct biomechanical issues, and alleviate symptoms.

- Metatarsal pads: Placing metatarsal pads or cushions under the ball of the foot can help spread the metatarsal heads and relieve pressure on the affected nerves.

- Padding and taping: Applying foam padding or felt cushions around the affected area or taping the toes

to maintain proper alignment and reduce friction and irritation.

- Medications: Nonsteroidal anti-inflammatory drugs (NSAIDs) such as ibuprofen or naproxen may be used to alleviate pain and inflammation associated with Morton's neuroma.

- Corticosteroid injections: Injections of corticosteroids into the affected area can help reduce inflammation and provide temporary relief of symptoms. However, repeated injections should be avoided due to the risk of tissue damage and nerve atrophy.

- Physical therapy: Modalities such as ultrasound, laser therapy, or electrical stimulation may be used to promote tissue healing and reduce pain. Stretching and strengthening exercises may also be prescribed to improve foot mechanics and reduce stress on the nerves.

- Alcohol sclerosing injections: Injections of alcohol or other sclerosing agents into the neuroma may be considered to reduce its size and relieve symptoms. This treatment is typically reserved for cases that do not respond to conservative measures.

- Extracorporeal shock wave therapy (ESWT): A noninvasive treatment modality that uses shock waves to stimulate healing and reduce pain in chronic cases of Morton's neuroma.

- Surgical intervention: In cases of severe or refractory Morton's neuroma that do not respond to conservative treatments, surgical procedures such as neuroma excision, nerve decompression, or neurectomy may be considered to remove the affected nerve tissue and alleviate symptoms.

6. Complications and Prognosis: With appropriate treatment, most cases of Morton's neuroma can be effectively managed, and symptoms can be relieved. However, untreated or recurrent cases of Morton's neuroma can lead to chronic pain, nerve damage, altered foot mechanics, and decreased mobility. Complications of Morton's neuroma may include persistent pain, sensory loss, gait abnormalities, foot deformities, and decreased quality of life. Early intervention, proper footwear, and modification of risk factors are essential for optimizing outcomes and preventing long-term complications in individuals with Morton's neuroma.

Morton's neuroma is a painful condition characterized by thickening of the tissue around the nerves between the toes. Prompt diagnosis, conservative management, and modification of contributing factors are key to effective treatment and prevention of complications. Individuals experiencing symptoms suggestive of Morton's neuroma should seek evaluation and guidance from a healthcare professional for an accurate diagnosis and individualized treatment plan.

8. TARSAL TUNNEL SYNDROME

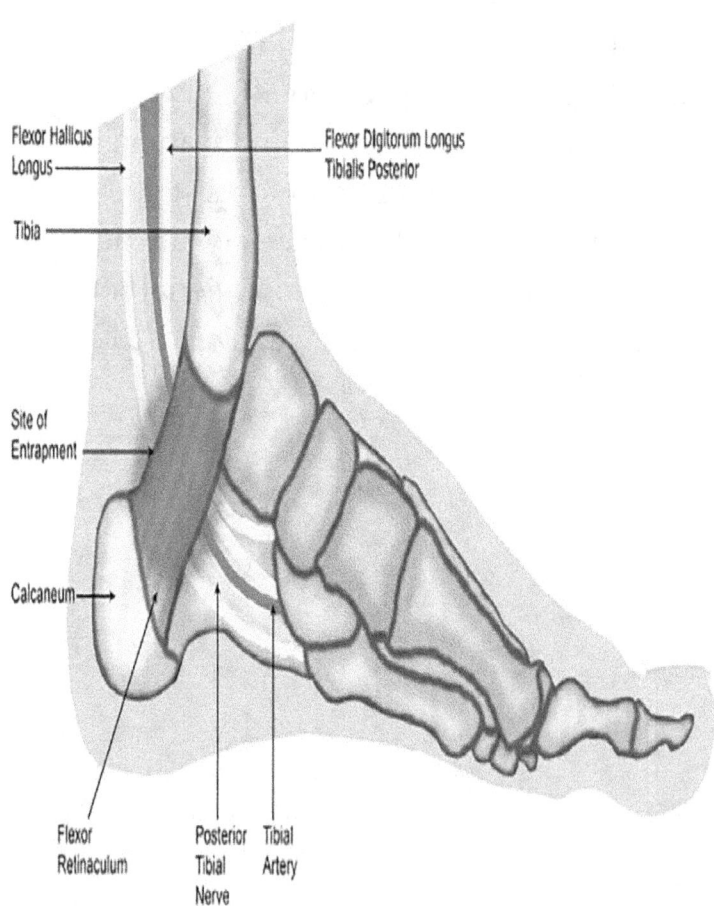

Flexor Hallicus Longus

Flexor Digitorum Longus
Tibialis Posterior

Tibia

Site of Entrapment

Calcaneum

Flexor Retinaculum

Posterior Tibial Nerve

Tibial Artery

Tarsal tunnel syndrome (TTS) is a painful condition caused by compression or irritation of the tibial nerve as it passes through the tarsal tunnel, a narrow space located on the inside of the ankle. This compression can lead to symptoms such as pain, tingling, burning sensations, and numbness in the foot and ankle. Tarsal tunnel syndrome is analogous to carpal tunnel syndrome but affects the lower extremity rather than the wrist.

Here's an extremely detailed overview of tarsal tunnel syndrome:

1. Anatomy of the Tarsal Tunnel: The tarsal tunnel is a narrow space located on the inside of the ankle, formed by the bones of the ankle (medial malleolus), the flexor retinaculum (a thick band of tissue that spans the ankle), and various tendons and ligaments. Within the tarsal tunnel, the tibial nerve, along with blood vessels and tendons, passes from the leg into the foot. The tibial nerve provides sensory innervation to

the bottom of the foot and motor function to
certain muscles of the foot and lower leg.

2. Causes of Tarsal Tunnel Syndrome: Tarsal
tunnel syndrome can occur due to various factors
that compress or irritate the tibial nerve as it
passes through the tarsal tunnel. Common causes
include:
   - Anatomical variations: Abnormalities in foot
structure, such as flat feet, high arches, or bony
prominences, can narrow the tarsal tunnel and
increase pressure on the tibial nerve.
   - Trauma or injury: Direct trauma to the ankle,
such as fractures, sprains, or crush injuries, can
cause swelling or scar tissue formation within
the tarsal tunnel, leading to nerve compression.
   - Overuse or repetitive stress: Activities that
involve repetitive ankle movements, such as
running, walking, or standing for prolonged
periods, can irritate the tibial nerve and
exacerbate symptoms.
   - Systemic conditions: Certain systemic
diseases or medical conditions, such as diabetes,
rheumatoid arthritis, hypothyroidism, or obesity,

can predispose individuals to nerve compression and tarsal tunnel syndrome.

- Space-occupying lesions: Benign or malignant tumors, ganglion cysts, varicose veins, or inflamed tendons within the tarsal tunnel can compress the tibial nerve and cause symptoms of tarsal tunnel syndrome.

- Pregnancy: Hormonal changes and weight gain during pregnancy can increase pressure on the tarsal tunnel and exacerbate symptoms in some individuals.

3. Symptoms of Tarsal Tunnel Syndrome: The symptoms of tarsal tunnel syndrome can vary in severity and may worsen over time. Common signs and symptoms may include:

- Pain or discomfort along the inside of the ankle or the bottom of the foot, radiating into the toes or the arch of the foot.

- Tingling, burning, or electric shock-like sensations in the foot and toes.

- Numbness or loss of sensation in the sole of the foot or toes.

- Weakness or muscle atrophy in the foot or toes.
- Symptoms that worsen with activity or prolonged standing and improve with rest or elevation of the foot.
- Tenderness or swelling along the course of the tarsal tunnel.

4. Diagnosis of Tarsal Tunnel Syndrome:
Diagnosing tarsal tunnel syndrome typically involves a combination of medical history, physical examination, and diagnostic tests. Common methods used to diagnose tarsal tunnel syndrome include:
- Medical history: A healthcare professional will inquire about symptoms, medical conditions, medications, previous injuries, and activity level.
- Physical examination: Assessment of the foot and ankle for signs of tenderness, swelling, or muscle weakness, as well as evaluation of foot structure, gait mechanics, and range of motion.
- Tinel's sign: A diagnostic maneuver where the healthcare professional taps or applies

pressure to the tarsal tunnel, causing tingling or electric shock-like sensations in the foot.

- Compression test: Compression of the tarsal tunnel with the thumb or fingers to reproduce symptoms and elicit tenderness along the course of the tibial nerve.

- Nerve conduction studies: Electrophysiological tests that measure the speed and amplitude of nerve impulses along the tibial nerve to assess for nerve dysfunction or damage.

- Imaging studies: X-rays, ultrasound, MRI scans, or CT scans may be ordered to visualize the anatomy of the foot and ankle, rule out other potential causes of symptoms, and identify space-occupying lesions or structural abnormalities within the tarsal tunnel.

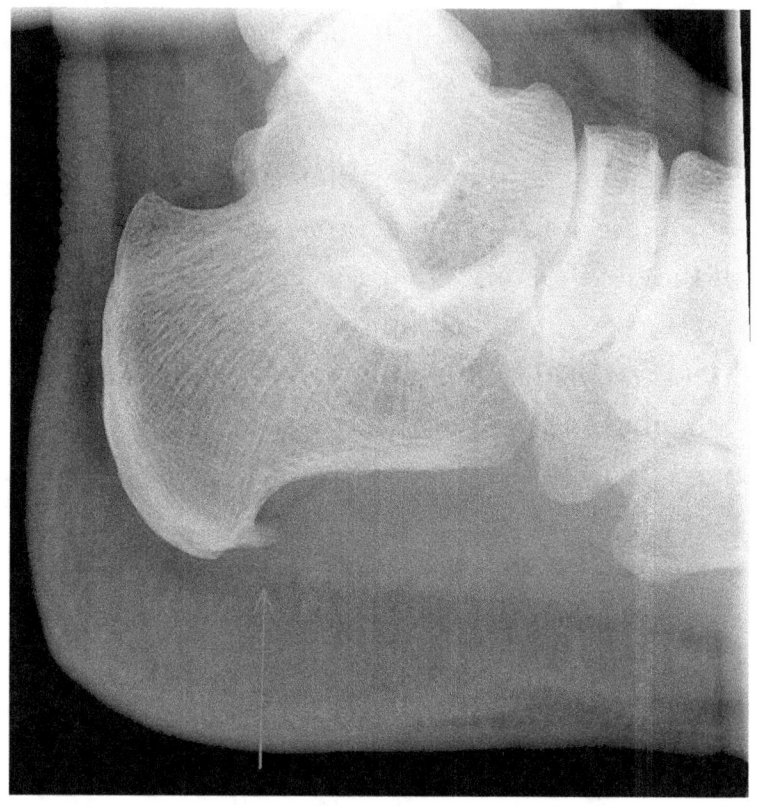

5. Treatment of Tarsal Tunnel Syndrome: Treatment for tarsal tunnel syndrome aims to relieve pain, reduce inflammation, and alleviate pressure on the tibial nerve. Depending on the severity of symptoms and underlying causes, treatment options may include:

- Rest and activity modification: Avoiding activities that exacerbate symptoms and providing adequate rest for the affected foot to heal.
- Orthotic devices: Custom orthotic inserts, arch supports, or night splints may be prescribed to redistribute pressure on the foot, correct foot mechanics, and alleviate symptoms.
- Footwear modifications: Wearing supportive

, well-fitting shoes with cushioned insoles and low heels to reduce pressure on the tarsal tunnel and provide shock absorption.
- Medications: Nonsteroidal anti-inflammatory drugs (NSAIDs) such as ibuprofen or naproxen may be used to alleviate pain and inflammation associated with tarsal tunnel syndrome.
- Corticosteroid injections: Injections of corticosteroids into the tarsal tunnel can help reduce inflammation and provide temporary relief of symptoms. However, repeated injections should be avoided due to the risk of tissue damage and nerve atrophy.

- Physical therapy: Modalities such as ultrasound, laser therapy, or electrical stimulation may be used to promote tissue healing and reduce pain. Stretching and strengthening exercises may also be prescribed to improve foot mechanics, increase flexibility, and reduce nerve compression.

- Nerve decompression surgery: In cases of severe or refractory tarsal tunnel syndrome that do not respond to conservative treatments, surgical decompression of the tarsal tunnel may be necessary to release pressure on the tibial nerve and alleviate symptoms. During surgery, the flexor retinaculum may be cut or released to create more space within the tarsal tunnel and relieve compression on the nerve.

6. Complications and Prognosis: With appropriate treatment, most cases of tarsal tunnel syndrome can be effectively managed, and symptoms can be relieved. However, untreated or recurrent cases of tarsal tunnel syndrome can lead to chronic pain, nerve damage, muscle weakness, altered foot mechanics, and decreased

mobility. Complications of tarsal tunnel syndrome may include persistent symptoms, sensory loss, motor deficits, gait abnormalities, and decreased quality of life. Early intervention, proper footwear, and modification of risk factors are essential for optimizing outcomes and preventing long-term complications in individuals with tarsal tunnel syndrome.

tarsal tunnel syndrome is a painful condition caused by compression or irritation of the tibial nerve as it passes through the tarsal tunnel. Prompt diagnosis, conservative management, and modification of contributing factors are key to effective treatment and prevention of complications. Individuals experiencing symptoms suggestive of tarsal tunnel syndrome should seek evaluation and guidance from a healthcare professional for an accurate diagnosis and individualized treatment plan.

9. BURSITIS

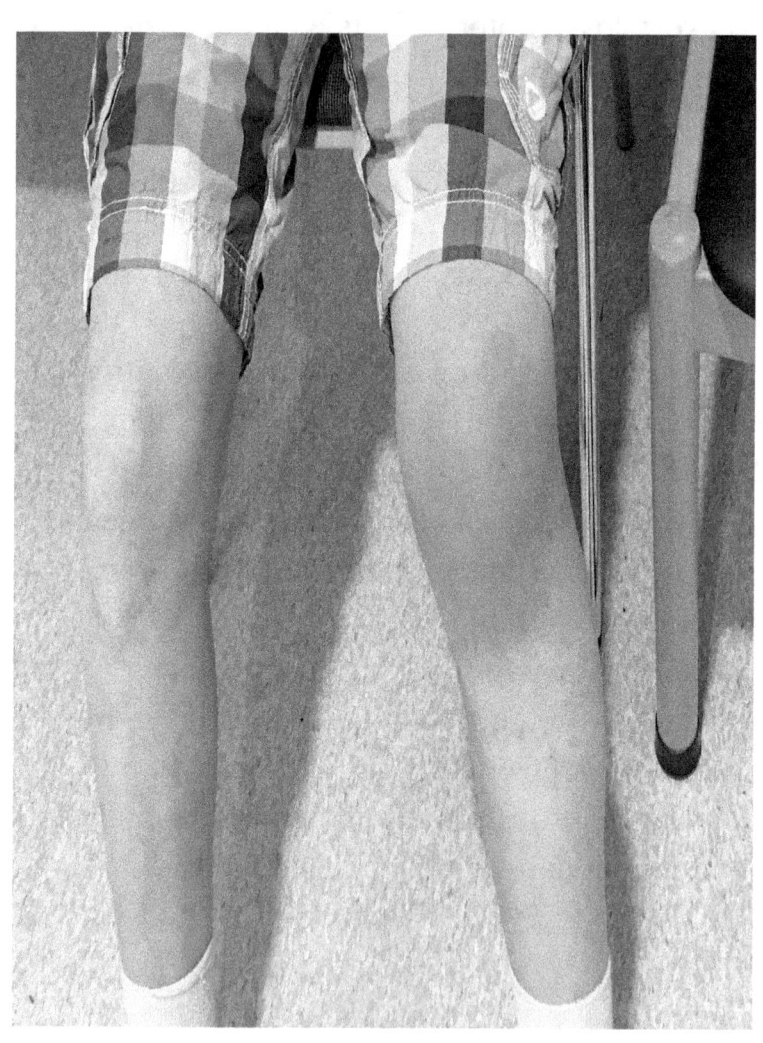

Bursitis is a painful condition characterized by inflammation or irritation of the bursae, small fluid-filled sacs located throughout the body near joints and between tendons and bones. These bursae serve to reduce friction and cushion the movement of muscles, tendons, and bones during movement. When bursae become inflamed or irritated, usually due to repetitive movements, trauma, or underlying medical conditions, it can lead to pain, swelling, and limited mobility in the affected joint.

Here's an extremely detailed overview of bursitis:

1. Anatomy of Bursae: Bursae are small, fluid-filled sacs lined with synovial membrane and filled with synovial fluid, located near joints throughout the body. They serve to reduce friction and cushion the movement of muscles, tendons, and bones during movement. Bursae are strategically positioned in areas prone to repetitive motion or pressure, such as the shoulders, elbows, hips, knees, and heels.

2. Types of Bursitis: Bursitis can occur in various locations throughout the body, depending on the affected bursae and underlying causes. Common types of bursitis include:

- Subacromial bursitis: Inflammation of the bursa located beneath the acromion process of the shoulder blade, often associated with shoulder impingement syndrome or rotator cuff injuries.

- Olecranon bursitis: Inflammation of the bursa located at the tip of the elbow (olecranon), commonly known as "student's elbow" or "miner's elbow."

- Trochanteric bursitis: Inflammation of the bursa located on the outside of the hip, over the greater trochanter of the femur, often associated with hip abductor tendonitis or iliotibial band syndrome.

- Prepatellar bursitis: Inflammation of the bursa located in front of the kneecap (patella), also known as "housemaid's knee."

- Retrocalcaneal bursitis: Inflammation of the bursa located at the back of the heel (retrocalcaneal), often associated with Achilles tendonitis or Haglund's deformity.

- Ischial bursitis: Inflammation of the bursa located between the hamstring muscles and the sitting bones (ischial tuberosities), commonly known as "weaver's bottom" or "driver's bottom."

- Plantar calcaneal bursitis: Inflammation of the bursa located beneath the heel bone (calcaneus), often associated with plantar fasciitis or heel spurs.

3. Causes of Bursitis: Bursitis can develop due to various factors that cause irritation, inflammation, or increased pressure on the bursae. Common causes include:

- Repetitive motion: Activities or occupations that involve repetitive movements or prolonged pressure on specific joints, such as overhead lifting, gardening, typing, kneeling, or running, can lead to bursitis.

- Trauma or injury: Direct trauma or blows to the affected joint, falls, or sudden impact injuries can cause inflammation of the bursae and lead to bursitis.

- Poor posture or biomechanics: Incorrect lifting techniques, improper body mechanics, or abnormal joint alignment can increase stress on the bursae and predispose individuals to bursitis.

- Overuse or excessive training: Engaging in high-intensity or repetitive physical activities without proper warm-up, cooldown, or rest periods can strain the muscles, tendons, and bursae, leading to bursitis.

- Medical conditions: Underlying medical conditions such as rheumatoid arthritis, gout, diabetes, thyroid disorders, or infections can increase the risk of bursitis due to inflammation, metabolic disturbances, or compromised immune function.

- Age-related changes: Degenerative changes in joint structures, reduced flexibility, or loss of muscle mass with aging can contribute to bursitis and other musculoskeletal disorders.

4. Symptoms of Bursitis: The symptoms of bursitis can vary depending on the location and

severity of inflammation. Common signs and symptoms may include:

- Pain or tenderness in the affected joint, typically worsened with movement or pressure and relieved with rest.

- Swelling, warmth, or redness around the affected area, indicating inflammation of the bursae.

- Stiffness or limited range of motion in the affected joint, especially during activities that involve bending, lifting, or bearing weight.

- Crepitus or crackling sensation with joint movement in some cases.

- Difficulty with activities such as lifting, reaching, climbing stairs, or kneeling, depending on the location of bursitis.

- Symptoms that worsen at night or with prolonged periods of immobility.

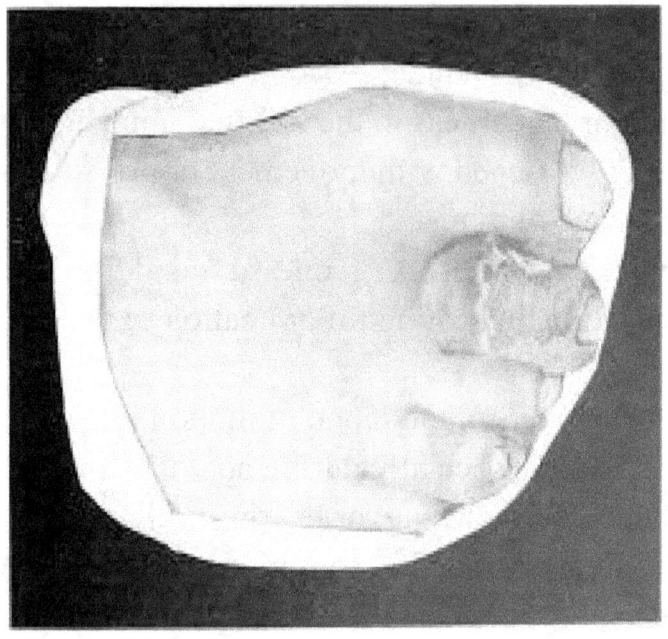

5. Diagnosis of Bursitis: Diagnosing bursitis typically involves a combination of medical history, physical examination, and diagnostic tests. Common methods used to diagnose bursitis include:

- Medical history: A healthcare professional will inquire about symptoms, onset, duration, exacerbating factors, medical conditions, medications, and previous injuries or activities.

- Physical examination: Assessment of the affected joint for signs of tenderness, swelling, warmth, or limited range of motion, as well as evaluation of posture, gait, and muscle strength.

- Palpation: Gentle palpation of the affected area to elicit tenderness, reproduce symptoms, and identify the location of inflammation or swelling.

- Range of motion testing: Assessment of joint flexibility, strength, and stability, as well as observation of functional movements to identify limitations or compensatory patterns.

- Imaging studies: X-rays, ultrasound, MRI scans, or CT scans may be ordered to visualize the anatomy of the affected joint, rule out other potential causes of symptoms, and assess for signs of bursitis, such as fluid accumulation or soft tissue abnormalities.

6. Treatment of Bursitis: Treatment for bursitis aims to relieve pain, reduce inflammation, and promote healing of the affected bursae. Depending on the location and severity of symptoms, treatment options may include:

- Rest and activity modification: Avoiding activities that exacerbate symptoms and providing adequate rest for the affected joint to heal.

- Ice therapy: Applying ice packs to the affected area for 15-20 minutes several times a day to reduce pain and inflammation.

- Compression: Using compression bandages or sleeves to reduce swelling and support the affected joint during activities.

- Elevation: Keeping the affected limb elevated above the level of the heart to reduce swelling and promote drainage of fluid from the affected area.

- Nonsteroidal anti-inflammatory drugs (NSAIDs): Oral medications such as ibuprofen or naproxen may be used to alleviate pain and inflammation associated with bursitis.

- Corticosteroid injections: Injections of corticosteroids into the affected bursae can help reduce inflammation and provide temporary relief of symptoms. However, repeated injections should be avoided due to the risk of tissue damage and systemic side effects.

- Physical therapy: Modalities such as ultrasound, laser therapy, or electrical stimulation may be used to promote tissue healing and reduce pain. Stretching and strengthening exercises may also be prescribed to improve joint mobility, stability, and function.

- Occupational therapy: Techniques to optimize ergonomics, joint protection, and energy

 conservation during daily activities may be taught to individuals with chronic or recurrent bursitis.

- Aspiration and drainage: In cases of severe or symptomatic fluid accumulation within the bursae, aspiration or drainage of the fluid may be performed under sterile conditions to alleviate pain and reduce swelling.

- Surgical intervention: In rare cases of severe or refractory bursitis that do not respond to conservative treatments, surgical procedures such as bursectomy (removal of the affected bursa) may be considered to alleviate symptoms and prevent recurrence.

7. Complications and Prognosis: With appropriate treatment, most cases of bursitis can be effectively managed, and symptoms can be relieved. However, untreated or recurrent cases of bursitis can lead to chronic pain, joint stiffness, muscle weakness, altered biomechanics, and decreased quality of life. Complications of bursitis may include persistent symptoms, recurrent flare-ups, joint instability, and increased risk of secondary injuries. Early intervention, proper biomechanics, and modification of risk factors are essential for optimizing outcomes and preventing long-term complications in individuals with bursitis.

 bursitis is a painful condition characterized by inflammation or irritation of the bursae, small fluid-filled sacs located throughout the body near joints. Prompt diagnosis, conservative management, and modification of contributing factors are key to effective treatment and prevention of complications. Individuals experiencing symptoms suggestive of bursitis should seek evaluation and guidance from a healthcare professional for an accurate diagnosis and individualized treatment plan.

10. GOUT

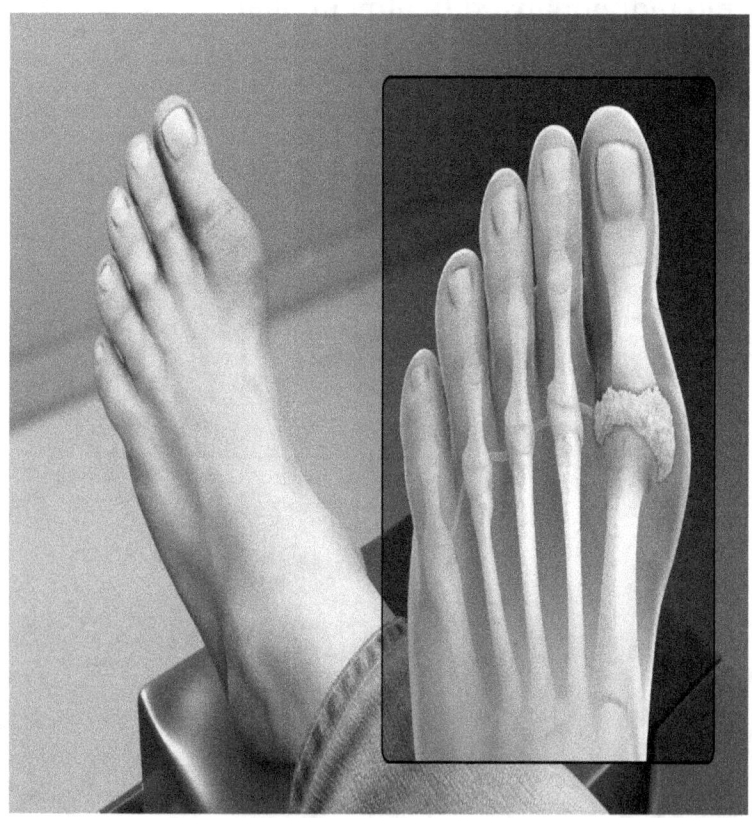

Gout is a complex form of inflammatory arthritis characterized by sudden and severe attacks of pain, swelling, redness, and tenderness in the joints, often affecting the big toe initially. It is caused by the buildup of uric acid crystals in the joints and surrounding tissues, leading to inflammation and debilitating symptoms. Gout attacks can be excruciatingly painful and may occur sporadically or become chronic if left untreated.

Here's an extremely detailed overview of gout:

1. Pathophysiology of Gout: Gout is primarily caused by hyperuricemia, a condition characterized by elevated levels of uric acid in the blood. Uric acid is a waste product formed during the breakdown of purines, compounds found in certain foods and beverages, as well as produced naturally by the body. When uric acid levels exceed the body's capacity to excrete it through the kidneys, it can accumulate in the bloodstream and form needle-like crystals of monosodium urate, which deposit in the joints and soft tissues, triggering an inflammatory response. The deposition of urate crystals leads to acute gout attacks, chronic inflammation, and progressive joint damage if left untreated.

2. Risk Factors for Gout: Several factors can increase the risk of developing gout, including:

- Genetics: Family history of gout or inherited conditions that affect uric acid metabolism, such as familial juvenile hyperuricemic nephropathy or Lesch-Nyhan syndrome.

- Diet: Consumption of purine-rich foods and beverages, such as red meat, organ meats, seafood, beer, and sugary drinks, can increase uric acid production and contribute to gout.

- Lifestyle factors: Obesity, sedentary lifestyle, excessive alcohol consumption, dehydration, and stress can exacerbate hyperuricemia and trigger gout attacks.

- Medical conditions: Chronic kidney disease, hypertension, metabolic syndrome, diabetes, cardiovascular disease, and certain medications (e.g., diuretics, aspirin, immunosuppressants) can impair uric acid excretion and predispose individuals to gout.

- Age and gender: Gout is more common in men than women, with onset typically occurring after puberty in males and after menopause in females. Risk increases with age, particularly in men over 40 and women over 60.

3. Clinical Manifestations of Gout: Gout typically presents with acute episodes of intense joint pain, swelling, redness, and warmth, commonly affecting the big toe (podagra) initially, although other joints such as the ankles, knees, wrists, and elbows may also be involved. Gout attacks often occur suddenly, often at night or in the early morning, and can last for days to weeks if left untreated. In between attacks, some individuals may experience periods of remission with no symptoms, while others may develop chronic gout characterized by persistent low-grade inflammation and joint damage. Chronic gout can lead to tophi, visible deposits of urate crystals beneath the skin, as well as joint deformities, joint erosion, and functional impairment.

4. Diagnosis of Gout: Diagnosing gout involves a combination of clinical assessment, medical history, physical examination, laboratory tests,

and imaging studies. Common methods used to diagnose gout include:

- Medical history: A healthcare professional will inquire about symptoms, onset, duration, frequency, severity, triggers, medical conditions, medications, diet, alcohol intake, family history, and lifestyle factors.

- Physical examination: Assessment of the affected joint(s) for signs of inflammation, tenderness, swelling, redness, and warmth, as well as evaluation of joint range of motion, gait, and functional status.

- Laboratory tests: Measurement of serum uric acid levels to assess for hyperuricemia, although levels may be normal during acute attacks. Synovial fluid analysis via joint aspiration to identify urate crystals under polarized light microscopy, which confirms the diagnosis of gout.

- Imaging studies: X-rays, ultrasound, or CT scans may be ordered to visualize joint structures, assess for joint damage or tophi, and rule out other potential causes of joint pain, such as infection or osteoarthritis.

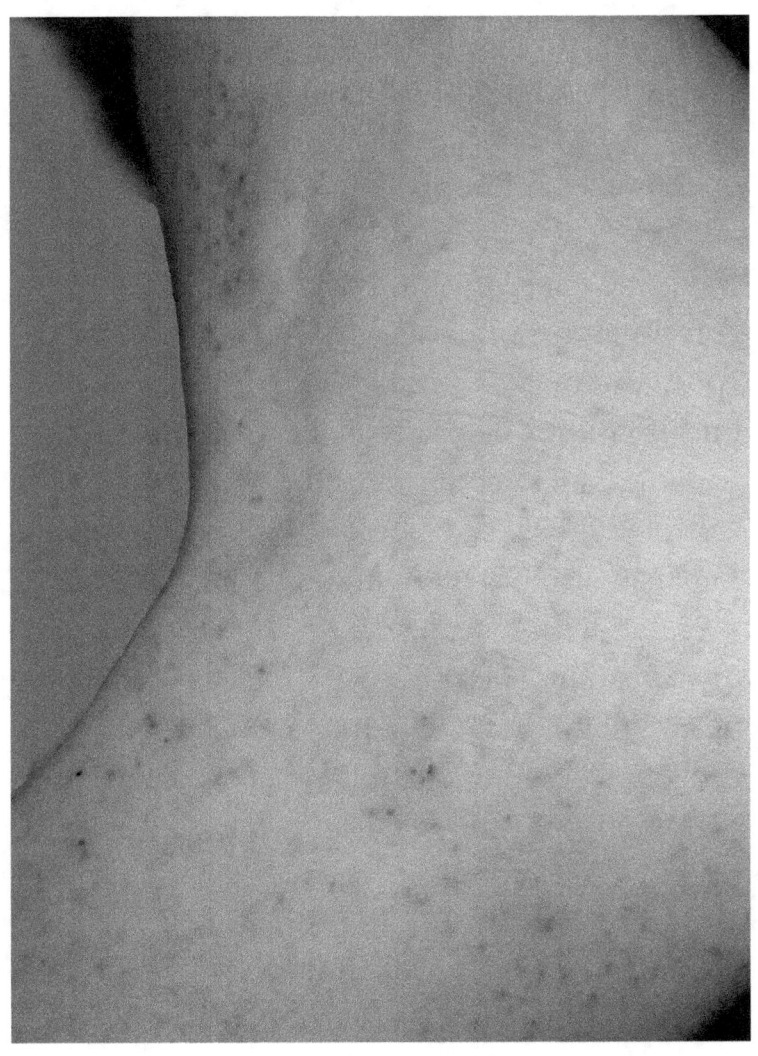

5. Treatment of Gout: Treatment for gout aims to relieve symptoms, reduce inflammation, lower uric acid levels, prevent acute attacks, and minimize long-term complications. Depending on the severity and stage of gout, treatment options may include:

- Acute management: Nonsteroidal anti-inflammatory drugs (NSAIDs), colchicine, corticosteroids, or intra-articular steroid injections may be prescribed to alleviate pain and inflammation during acute gout attacks. Rest, ice packs, and elevation of the affected joint can also provide symptomatic relief.

- Long-term management: Lifestyle modifications such as dietary changes (reducing purine-rich foods, alcohol intake, and sugary drinks), weight loss, regular exercise, adequate hydration, and stress management to lower uric acid levels and prevent gout flares.

- Medications: Urate-lowering therapy (ULT) medications such as allopurinol, febuxostat, or probenecid may be prescribed to decrease uric acid production or increase uric acid excretion and prevent recurrent gout attacks. Medications such as pegloticase or lesinurad may be considered for refractory cases or individuals with severe gout.

- Colchicine prophylaxis: Low-dose colchicine or NSAIDs may be prescribed during initiation of ULT or after acute gout attacks to prevent flare-ups.

- Tophi management: Surgical excision, aspiration, or dissolution therapy (e.g., oral or intralesional corticosteroids, febuxostat, or pegloticase) may be considered for tophi that are painful, recurrent, or cosmetically bothersome.

- Patient education: Providing information about gout triggers, lifestyle modifications, medication adherence, and self-management strategies to empower individuals to manage their condition effectively and prevent complications.

6. Complications and Prognosis: With appropriate treatment and lifestyle modifications, most cases of gout can be effectively managed, and symptoms can be controlled. However, untreated or poorly

managed gout can lead to chronic pain, joint damage, deformities, functional impairment, and decreased quality of life. Complications of gout may include recurrent acute attacks, chronic inflammation, joint erosions, tophi formation, nephrolithiasis (kidney stones), nephropathy, cardiovascular disease, and metabolic syndrome. Early intervention, regular monitoring, and modification of risk

 factors are essential for optimizing outcomes and preventing long-term complications in individuals with gout.

gout is a painful and debilitating form of inflammatory arthritis caused by the buildup of uric acid crystals in the joints and surrounding tissues. Prompt diagnosis, aggressive treatment of acute attacks, and long-term management to lower uric acid levels are crucial for controlling symptoms, preventing recurrence, and minimizing joint damage in individuals with gout. Individuals experiencing symptoms suggestive of gout should seek evaluation and guidance from a healthcare professional for an accurate diagnosis and individualized treatment plan.

www.ingramcontent.com/pod-product-compliance
Lightning Source LLC
Chambersburg PA
CBHW071056290526
45795CB00004B/1513